POLLEN ALLERGY: THE ESSENTIAL HANDBOOK TO BREAK FREE FROM POLLEN ALLERGY SEASON

DR.PETE

POLLEN ALLERGY

CONTENTS

INTRODUCTION

Are you tired of sneezing fits, itchy eyes, and congestion every time spring arrives?

Do you dread the sight of blooming flowers and trees, knowing that it means weeks or even months of discomfort and frustration? If so, you're not alone.

Pollen allergies affect millions of people worldwide, making seasonal changes a dreaded time rather than a cause for celebration.

Pollen allergies, also known as hay fever or allergic rhinitis, can turn the most beautiful of seasons into a nightmare for sufferers. Imagine trying to enjoy a picnic in the park or a leisurely stroll through the countryside, only to be overwhelmed by relentless sneezing and a constant stream of tissues.

Picture waking up every morning with puffy eyes and a stuffy nose, feeling like you've barely slept at all. Consider the impact on your work, your social life, and your overall well-being when every breath feels like a battle against nature itself.

But fear not, relief is within reach. In this essential handbook, we'll explore everything you need to know to break free from the grip of pollen allergy season. From understanding the root causes of your symptoms to implementing practical strategies for managing and minimizing your exposure to pollen, this book is your comprehensive guide to reclaiming control over your health and your life.

By arming yourself with knowledge and adopting proactive measures, you can turn allergy season from a time of dread into an opportunity for empowerment and renewal. It's time to say goodbye to sneezing fits and itchy eyes and hello to a brighter, allergy-free future.

Understanding Pollen Allergies

What is Pollen?

Pollen, often associated with the beauty of blossoming flowers and the vitality of spring, is actually a common trigger for allergic reactions in many individuals. It is a fine, powdery substance produced via way of means of flowers as a part of their reproductive process.. While essential for plant reproduction, pollen can wreak havoc on the respiratory systems of allergy sufferers when inhaled.

How Pollen Allergies Develop

Pollen allergies, also known as hay fever or allergic rhinitis, occur when the immune system mistakenly identifies pollen as a threat and mounts an exaggerated response to protect the body. This hypersensitivity leads to the release of histamines and other inflammatory substances, causing the characteristic symptoms of allergic reactions.

Common Symptoms of Pollen Allergies

The symptoms of pollen allergies can vary in severity from mild to debilitating and may include:
- Sneezing
- Runny or stuffy nose
- Itchy or watery eyes
- Nasal congestion
- Postnasal drip
- Coughing
- Fatigue
- Headache
- Itchy throat or ears

These symptoms can significantly impact daily life, interfering with work, school, and leisure activities.

Understanding the nature of pollen allergies and their symptoms is the first step toward effectively managing and mitigating their effects on your health and well-being.

In the chapters that follow, we will delve deeper into the intricacies of pollen allergies and explore strategies for finding relief and reclaiming control over your life during pollen allergy season.

Chapter 1: Identifying Your Triggers

Pollen allergies are not a one-size-fits-all condition; they vary depending on the specific types of pollen to which an individual is allergic.

In this chapter, we'll delve into the diverse world of pollen allergens, explore their seasonal patterns, and uncover the phenomenon of allergic cross-reactivity.

Types of Pollen Allergens

Imagine walking through a picturesque park, surrounded by majestic trees swaying in the breeze. While this scene may evoke feelings of tranquility for some, for others, it could trigger a torrent of sneezes and itchy eyes. **Tree pollen**, produced by a variety of tree species including oak, birch, and cedar, is a common culprit behind springtime allergies. Each tree species releases its pollen at different times throughout the year, contributing to the complexity of seasonal allergies.

But trees are not the only source of pollen allergies; grasses also play a significant role. Picture the sprawling green lawns of summertime, inviting you to kick off your shoes and revel in the warmth of the sun. For those sensitive to **grass pollen**, however, this idyllic scene may be marred by relentless symptoms of allergic rhinitis. Grass pollen allergies are particularly prevalent during the late spring and early summer months when grasses are in full bloom.

As if tree and grass pollen weren't enough to contend with, **weed pollen** adds another layer of complexity to the allergen landscape. Weeds such as ragweed, sagebrush, and pigweed release their pollen in late summer and early fall, extending the allergy season well into the cooler months.

Recognizing Seasonal Patterns

Understanding the seasonal patterns of pollen allergens is essential for managing allergy symptoms effectively. By keeping track of when specific allergens are most prevalent in your area, you can take proactive measures to minimize your exposure and alleviate symptoms.

For example, if you know that tree pollen tends to peak in early spring, you might choose to spend more time indoors or wear a protective mask when outdoors during that time.

Allergic Cross-Reactivity

Allergic cross-reactivity, also known as pollen-food syndrome or oral allergy syndrome, is a fascinating yet often overlooked aspect of pollen allergies. This phenomenon occurs when proteins in certain fruits, vegetables, or nuts resemble the proteins found in pollen, leading to an allergic reaction in individuals with pollen allergies. For instance, someone allergic to birch pollen may experience oral itching or swelling after eating apples or cherries, which contain similar proteins.

By identifying your specific pollen triggers, recognizing seasonal patterns, and understanding the concept of allergic cross-reactivity, you can take proactive steps to manage your pollen allergies more effectively. In the chapters that follow, we'll explore strategies for minimizing exposure to pollen and finding relief from allergy symptoms year-round.

Chapter 2: Diagnosis and Testing

For many individuals suffering from pollen allergies, the journey to finding relief begins with a proper diagnosis. In this chapter, we'll explore the importance of consulting with healthcare professionals, the various allergy testing options available, and how to understand the results of these tests. By taking these steps, you can gain valuable insights into your allergy triggers and develop a personalized plan for managing your symptoms effectively.

Consulting with Healthcare Professionals

Imagine you've been experiencing persistent symptoms of sneezing, nasal congestion, and itchy eyes every spring for as long as you can remember. Fed up with constantly reaching for tissues and over-the-counter allergy medications, you decide it's time to seek professional help. This decision marks the first step on your journey to understanding and managing your pollen allergies.

Consulting with a healthcare professional, such as an allergist or immunologist, is crucial for obtaining an accurate diagnosis and developing an effective treatment plan. During your initial consultation, your healthcare provider will conduct a thorough medical history review and may perform a physical examination to assess your symptoms and overall health.

Be prepared to provide detailed information about your allergy symptoms, including when they occur, their duration and severity, and any factors that seem to trigger or worsen them. This information will help your healthcare provider form a comprehensive picture of your allergy profile and guide further diagnostic testing.

Allergy Testing Options

Once your healthcare provider has gathered sufficient information about your symptoms and medical history, they may recommend allergy testing to identify specific allergens that are triggering your symptoms. There are numerous sorts of allergic reaction checks available, with its personal benefits and limitations.

Skin prick testing, also known as puncture or scratch testing, is one of the most common methods used to diagnose pollen allergies. During this test, small amounts of common allergens, including tree, grass, and weed pollens, are applied to the skin's surface, usually on the forearm or back. The skin is then pricked or scratched to allow the allergens to penetrate the skin's barrier. If you are allergic to any of the substances tested, you will develop a small, raised bump or hive at the site of the allergen.

Another option for allergy testing is blood testing, also known as specific IgE testing. This involves drawing a blood sample and measuring the levels of specific antibodies, known as immunoglobulin E (IgE), that are produced in response to allergen exposure.

Blood testing can be particularly useful for individuals who cannot undergo skin prick testing due to certain medical conditions or medications.

In some cases, your healthcare provider may recommend patch testing to identify potential allergens that come into contact with your skin, such as certain cosmetics or topical medications. Patch testing involves applying small amounts of suspected allergens to patches placed on the skin's surface for a specified period, usually 48 hours. If you develop a reaction at the patch site, it indicates a sensitivity to the tested substance.

UNDERSTANDING TEST RESULTS

Once allergy testing has been completed, your healthcare provider will review the results with you and discuss their implications for your allergy management plan. It's essential to understand that a positive allergy test indicates sensitization to a specific allergen but does not necessarily mean that you will experience symptoms upon exposure. Conversely, a negative allergy test does not rule out the possibility of allergy symptoms.

Your healthcare provider will consider the results of allergy testing in conjunction with your medical history and symptoms to formulate a personalized treatment plan tailored to your individual needs. This may include allergen avoidance strategies, medication management, and, in some cases, allergen immunotherapy to desensitize your immune system to pollen allergens over time.

By consulting with healthcare professionals, undergoing appropriate allergy testing, and understanding the results, you can take proactive steps toward managing your pollen allergies effectively.

In the following chapters, we'll explore various strategies for minimizing your exposure to pollen and finding relief from allergy symptoms, allowing you to enjoy life to the fullest, even during pollen season.

Chapter 3: Managing Pollen Exposure

As pollen season approaches, many allergy sufferers brace themselves for the inevitable onslaught of symptoms. However, by implementing effective strategies to minimize exposure to pollen, you can significantly reduce the severity and frequency of allergic reactions.

In this chapter, we'll explore indoor allergen reduction strategies, outdoor allergy prevention techniques, and the use of pollen forecasting and monitoring tools to help you navigate pollen season with greater ease and comfort.

Indoor Allergen Reduction Strategies

Creating an allergy-friendly environment indoors is crucial for minimizing exposure to pollen and other airborne allergens. Consider the following strategies to reduce indoor allergens and create a sanctuary from pollen during allergy season:

1. Maintain a Clean Living Space: Regularly vacuuming carpets and upholstered furniture, dusting surfaces, and washing bedding in hot water can help remove pollen and other allergens from your home.

2. Use High-Efficiency Air Filters: Installing high-efficiency particulate air (HEPA) filters in your HVAC system and using HEPA air purifiers in key areas of your home can help trap pollen particles and improve indoor air quality.

3. Keep Windows Closed: During pollen season, keep windows and doors closed to prevent outdoor pollen from entering your home. Use air conditioning to maintain a comfortable indoor temperature without relying on open windows.

4. Limit Outdoor Clothing and Accessories: When returning home from outdoor activities, remove and wash outdoor clothing and accessories to prevent pollen from being tracked indoors.

5. Create a Pollen-Free Zone: Designate a specific area of your home, such as the bedroom, as a pollen-free zone by using allergen-proof pillow and mattress covers and keeping windows closed.

By implementing these indoor allergen reduction strategies, you can create a more comfortable living environment and minimize your exposure to pollen indoors.

Outdoor Allergy Prevention Techniques

While it's impossible to completely avoid outdoor pollen during allergy season, there are steps you can take to reduce your exposure and alleviate symptoms when spending time outdoors:

1. Check Pollen Counts: Before heading outdoors, check local pollen counts using online resources or mobile apps. Avoid spending extended periods outdoors on days when pollen counts are high.

2. Time Outdoor Activities Wisely: Pollen levels are typically highest in the early morning and early evening. Schedule outdoor activities for midday when pollen levels are lower.

3. Wear Protective Clothing: When spending time outdoors, wear long-sleeved shirts, pants, sunglasses, and a wide-brimmed hat to minimize skin and eye contact with pollen.

4. Use Pollen-Blocking Accessories: Consider using pollen-blocking accessories such as nasal filters or masks when gardening or engaging in outdoor activities during peak pollen season.

5. Shower and Change Clothes After Outdoor Activities: After spending time outdoors, shower and change into clean clothes to remove pollen from your skin and clothing.

By incorporating these outdoor allergy prevention techniques into your routine, you can enjoy outdoor activities with greater comfort and confidence during pollen season.

Pollen Forecasting and Monitoring Tools

Advances in technology have made it easier than ever to track pollen levels and make informed decisions about outdoor activities. Pollen forecasting and monitoring tools provide real-time information about pollen counts and allergen levels in your area, allowing you to plan accordingly and take steps to minimize exposure. Examples of pollen forecasting and monitoring tools include:

1. Pollen Count Apps: Mobile apps such as Pollen.com and AccuWeather offer pollen forecasts and allergy alerts based on your location, helping you stay informed about pollen levels in your area.

2. Online Pollen Trackers: Websites like the National Allergy Bureau (NAB) and Weather.com provide pollen count forecasts and maps, allowing you to visualize pollen levels and trends in your region.

3. Personal Pollen Monitors: Personal pollen monitors, such as the AeroTrak® Handheld Airborne Particle Counter, allow you to measure indoor and outdoor pollen levels in real-time, empowering you to make data-driven decisions about pollen exposure.

By utilizing pollen forecasting and monitoring tools, you can stay one step ahead of pollen season and take proactive measures to minimize exposure and manage your allergy symptoms effectively.

By implementing indoor allergen reduction strategies, outdoor allergy prevention techniques, and utilizing pollen forecasting and monitoring tools, you can take control of your pollen allergy symptoms and enjoy greater comfort and peace of mind during allergy season.

In the following chapters, we'll explore additional strategies for managing pollen allergies and finding relief from allergy symptoms.

CHAPTER 4: MEDICATIONS AND TREATMENTS

When it comes to managing pollen allergies, medications and treatments play a vital role in alleviating symptoms and improving quality of life.

In this chapter, we'll explore the various options available, including over-the-counter allergy medications, prescription allergy medications, and immunotherapy options, and how they can help you find relief from pollen allergy symptoms.

Over-the-Counter Allergy Medications

For many allergy sufferers, over-the-counter (OTC) allergy medications are the first line of defense against pollen allergy symptoms. These medications are readily available without a prescription and can help relieve common symptoms such as sneezing, itching, and nasal congestion. Some of the most common types of OTC allergy medications include:

1. Antihistamines: Antihistamines work by blocking the effects of histamine, a chemical released by the immune system in response to allergen exposure. Examples of OTC antihistamines include cetirizine (Zyrtec), loratadine (Claritin), and fexofenadine (Allegra).

2. Decongestants: Decongestants help relieve nasal congestion by narrowing blood vessels in the nasal passages, reducing swelling and congestion. Pseudoephedrine (Sudafed) and phenylephrine (Sudafed PE) are common decongestant ingredients found in OTC allergy medications.

3. Nasal Sprays: Nasal sprays containing corticosteroids, such as fluticasone (Flonase) and mometasone (Nasonex), help reduce inflammation and congestion in the nasal passages, providing relief from allergy symptoms.

4. Eye Drops: OTC eye drops containing antihistamines or mast cell stabilizers can help relieve itching, redness, and irritation caused by allergic conjunctivitis (allergic eye inflammation).

When using OTC allergy medications, it's essential to follow the manufacturer's instructions and consult with a healthcare professional if you have any questions or concerns about their use. While OTC medications can provide temporary relief from allergy symptoms, they may not address the underlying cause of your allergies.

Prescription Allergy Medications

For individuals with severe or persistent allergy symptoms, prescription allergy medications may be necessary to achieve adequate symptom control. Prescription allergy medications are typically stronger and more targeted than their OTC counterparts and may include:

1.   Intranasal   Corticosteroids: Prescription-strength   intranasal corticosteroid sprays, such as fluticasone (Flonase Sensimist) and budesonide (Rhinocort), are effective at reducing inflammation and congestion in the nasal passages, providing long-lasting relief from allergy symptoms.

2. Leukotriene Receptor Antagonists: Medications such as montelukast (Singulair) block the action of leukotrienes, inflammatory substances released by the immune system in response to allergen exposure. Leukotriene receptor antagonists can help relieve symptoms of allergic rhinitis and asthma.

3. Allergy Shots (Immunotherapy): Allergy shots, also known as allergen immunotherapy, involve administering gradually increasing doses of allergens to desensitize the immune system and reduce allergic reactions over time. This long-term treatment approach can be effective for individuals with severe allergies that do not respond to other treatments.

Before starting any prescription allergy medications, it's essential to consult with a healthcare professional to determine the most appropriate treatment plan for your specific allergy symptoms and medical history. Prescription allergy medications may have side effects and contraindications that should be carefully considered before use.

IMMUNOTHERAPY OPTIONS

For individuals with severe or persistent pollen allergies that do not respond to medication or allergen avoidance strategies, immunotherapy may offer long-term relief from symptoms. Immunotherapy, also known as allergy shots, works by gradually exposing the immune system to increasing doses of allergens, allowing the body to build tolerance over time. This process can help reduce allergic reactions and improve quality of life for allergy sufferers.

During immunotherapy treatment, allergy shots are administered at regular intervals, typically once or twice a week initially, and then gradually spaced out as tolerance develops. The duration of treatment varies depending on individual response and the severity of allergies but may last for several months to several years.

In addition to traditional allergy shots, sublingual immunotherapy (SLIT) tablets are also available for certain allergens, including grass and ragweed pollen. SLIT involves placing a tablet containing allergen extracts under the tongue and allowing it to dissolve, providing a convenient and effective alternative to allergy shots for some patients.

Immunotherapy is not suitable for everyone and may not be recommended for individuals with certain medical conditions or medication allergies. Before starting immunotherapy, it's essential to undergo thorough evaluation and consultation with an allergist or immunologist to determine eligibility and develop a personalized treatment plan.

By exploring the various medications and treatments available for pollen allergies, you can work with healthcare professionals to develop a comprehensive management plan tailored to your individual needs. Whether you opt for OTC allergy medications, prescription treatments, or immunotherapy, finding the right combination of therapies can help you achieve long-term relief from pollen allergy symptoms and improve your overall quality of life.

Chapter 5: Lifestyle Modifications

In addition to medications and treatments, lifestyle modifications play a crucial role in managing pollen allergies and reducing symptoms. In this chapter, we'll explore practical tips for creating an allergy-friendly home environment, dietary considerations for pollen allergy relief, and stress management techniques to help you navigate pollen season with greater ease and comfort.

ALLERGY-FRIENDLY HOME ENVIRONMENT TIPS

Your home should be a sanctuary from pollen and other allergens, providing a refuge where you can find relief from allergy symptoms. By implementing allergy-friendly home environment tips, you can create a space that promotes wellness and minimizes exposure to pollen. Consider the following strategies:

1. Minimize Indoor Plants: While indoor plants can improve air quality, they can also harbor pollen and other allergens. Opt for low-pollen plants such as spider plants, ferns, and succulents, and avoid high-pollen plants such as flowering trees and grasses.

2. Clean Regularly: Regular cleaning is essential for reducing indoor allergens such as dust, pet dander, and pollen. Vacuum carpets and upholstered furniture, dust surfaces, and wash bedding in hot water at least once a week to remove allergens from your home.

3. Use Air Purifiers: High-efficiency particulate air (HEPA) air purifiers can help remove pollen and other airborne allergens from indoor air, improving air quality and reducing allergy symptoms. Place air purifiers in key areas of your home, such as the bedroom and living room, for maximum effectiveness.

4. Keep Windows Closed: During pollen season, keep windows and doors closed to prevent outdoor pollen from entering your home. Use air conditioning to maintain a comfortable indoor temperature without relying on open windows.

5. Invest in Allergy-Proof Bedding: Allergen-proof pillow and mattress covers can help protect against dust mites, pollen, and other allergens, creating a barrier between you and potential triggers while you sleep.

By implementing these allergy-friendly home environment tips, you can create a comfortable and supportive living space that promotes wellness and minimizes exposure to pollen.

DIETARY CONSIDERATIONS FOR POLLEN ALLERGY RELIEF

While diet alone cannot cure pollen allergies, certain dietary considerations may help alleviate symptoms and support overall immune function. Incorporating anti-inflammatory foods, antioxidants, and nutrients into your diet can help reduce inflammation and strengthen your body's defenses against allergens. Consider the following dietary tips for pollen allergy relief:

1. Focus on Whole Foods: Choose a diet rich in whole foods such as fruits, vegetables, whole grains, lean protein sources, and healthy fats. These nutrient-dense foods provide essential vitamins, minerals, and antioxidants that support immune function and reduce inflammation.

2. Incorporate Omega-3 Fatty Acids: Omega-3 fatty acids, found in fatty fish, flaxseeds, chia seeds, and walnuts, have anti-inflammatory properties that may help reduce allergic inflammation and alleviate symptoms of pollen allergies.

3. Limit Pro-inflammatory Foods: Minimize your intake of pro-inflammatory foods such as refined sugars, processed foods, and trans fats, which can exacerbate allergic inflammation and weaken immune function.

4. Stay Hydrated: Drink plenty of water throughout the day to stay hydrated and support mucous membrane function. Adequate hydration helps maintain healthy nasal passages and reduces the risk of nasal congestion and irritation.

5. Consider Herbal Teas: Certain herbal teas, such as chamomile, nettle, and peppermint, have natural anti-inflammatory and antihistamine properties that may help alleviate allergy symptoms and promote relaxation.

While dietary considerations can complement other allergy management strategies, it's essential to consult with a healthcare professional before making significant changes to your diet, especially if you have underlying health conditions or food allergies.

STRESS MANAGEMENT TECHNIQUES

Stress can exacerbate allergy symptoms and weaken the immune system, making you more susceptible to allergic reactions. Incorporating stress management techniques into your daily routine can help reduce the impact of stress on your body and mind, improving your resilience to pollen allergies. Consider the following stress management techniques:

1. Practice Mindfulness Meditation: Mindfulness meditation involves focusing your attention on the present moment without judgment, allowing you to cultivate a sense of calm and relaxation. Spend a few minutes each day practicing mindfulness meditation to reduce stress and promote emotional well-being.

2. Engage in Physical Activity: Regular physical activity, such as walking, jogging, yoga, or tai chi, can help reduce stress levels and improve overall mood. Aim for at least 30 minutes of moderate-intensity exercise most days of the week to reap the benefits of physical activity for stress management.

3. Prioritize Self-Care: Take time for self-care activities that nourish your body and soul, such as taking a warm bath, reading a book, or spending time in nature. Engaging in sports that deliver you pleasure and rest can assist lessen pressure and enhance your universal well-being.

4. Practice Deep Breathing: Deep breathing exercises, such as diaphragmatic breathing or belly breathing, can help activate the body's relaxation response and reduce stress levels. Take slow, deep breaths in through your nose and out through your mouth, focusing on the sensation of your breath as it enters and leaves your body.

5. Seek Social Support: Reach out to friends, family members, or support groups for emotional support and connection. Sharing your experiences with others who understand can help reduce feelings of isolation and stress and provide a sense of belonging and community.

By incorporating these lifestyle modifications into your daily routine, you can create a supportive environment that promotes wellness and resilience during pollen season. From allergy-friendly home environment tips to dietary considerations and stress management techniques, finding what works best for you can help you navigate pollen season with greater ease and comfort.

In the following chapters, we'll explore additional strategies for managing pollen allergies and finding relief from allergy symptoms.

Chapter 6: Natural Remedies and Alternative Therapies

In addition to conventional medications and treatments, many individuals seek relief from pollen allergies through natural remedies and alternative therapies.

In this chapter, we'll explore the use of herbal supplements and remedies, acupuncture and acupressure, and breathing exercises and yoga as complementary approaches to managing pollen allergy symptoms..

Herbal Supplements and Remedies

Herbal supplements and remedies have been used for centuries to alleviate allergy symptoms and support overall health and wellness. While scientific evidence supporting the effectiveness of herbal remedies for pollen allergies is limited, some herbs may possess anti-inflammatory, antihistamine, and immune-modulating properties that could help reduce allergy symptoms. Consider the following herbal supplements and remedies commonly used for pollen allergy relief:

1. Butterbur: Butterbur extract, derived from the Petasites hybridus plant, has been studied for its potential effectiveness in relieving symptoms of allergic rhinitis, including sneezing, nasal congestion, and itching. Butterbur may work by inhibiting the release of histamine and other inflammatory substances in the body.

2. Quercetin: Quercetin is a flavonoid found in many fruits, vegetables, and herbs that has antioxidant and anti-inflammatory properties. Some research suggests that quercetin supplements may help reduce allergy symptoms by stabilizing mast cells and inhibiting the release of histamine.

3. Stinging Nettle: Stinging nettle (Urtica dioica) is a perennial plant that has been traditionally used to treat allergy symptoms, including hay fever and allergic rhinitis. Nettle extract may help reduce inflammation and nasal congestion associated with pollen allergies.

4. Bromelain: Bromelain is an enzyme found in pineapple that has anti-inflammatory properties and may help reduce swelling and inflammation in the nasal passages and sinuses. Bromelain supplements are sometimes used as a natural remedy for allergic rhinitis.

While herbal supplements and remedies may offer some relief from pollen allergy symptoms for some individuals, it's essential to consult with a healthcare professional before starting any new supplement regimen, particularly when you have underlying fitness situations or are taking medications..

ACUPUNCTURE AND ACUPRESSURE

Acupuncture and acupressure are traditional Chinese medicine techniques that involve stimulating specific points on the body to promote healing and relieve symptoms. While the scientific evidence supporting the effectiveness of acupuncture and acupressure for pollen allergies is mixed, some studies suggest that these techniques may help reduce allergy symptoms by modulating the immune response and promoting relaxation.

Acupuncture involves inserting thin needles into specific points on the body, known as acupuncture points, to stimulate energy flow and restore balance to the body's systems. Acupressure uses finger pressure on acupuncture points instead of needles to achieve similar therapeutic effects.

Some individuals find relief from pollen allergy symptoms through regular acupuncture or acupressure treatments, while others may not experience significant benefits. As with any alternative therapy, it's essential to consult with a qualified practitioner and discuss your treatment goals and expectations before starting acupuncture or acupressure for pollen allergies.

BREATHING EXERCISES AND YOGA

Breathing exercises and yoga techniques can help reduce stress, promote relaxation, and improve respiratory function, making them valuable tools for managing pollen allergy symptoms. Deep breathing exercises, such as diaphragmatic breathing or belly breathing, can help activate the body's relaxation response and reduce stress levels, which may help alleviate allergy symptoms.

Yoga combines bodily postures, respiration exercises, and meditation to promote average fitness and well-being.. Certain yoga poses, such as forward bends and twists, can help open up the chest and improve lung function, while relaxation techniques such as yoga nidra (yogic sleep) can promote deep relaxation and stress relief.

Practicing breathing exercises and yoga regularly during pollen season can help reduce the impact of allergy symptoms on your daily life and improve your overall quality of life. Consider incorporating these techniques into your daily routine to support your body's natural healing process and promote resilience during pollen season.

While natural remedies and alternative therapies may offer relief from pollen allergy symptoms for some individuals, it's essential to approach them with caution and consult with a healthcare professional before starting any new treatment regimen.

By combining conventional treatments with natural remedies and alternative therapies, you can develop a comprehensive approach to managing pollen allergies that addresses your individual needs and preferences.

In the following chapters, we'll explore additional strategies for managing pollen allergies and finding relief from allergy symptoms.

Chapter 7: Coping Strategies and Support

Living with pollen allergies can present unique challenges that extend beyond physical symptoms. In this chapter, we'll explore coping strategies for navigating emotional challenges, communicating with family, friends, and co-workers about your allergies, and finding support groups and resources to help you cope with pollen allergy season.

Navigating Emotional Challenges

Living with pollen allergies can take a toll on your emotional well-being, leading to feelings of frustration, isolation, and even anxiety or depression. It's essential to acknowledge and address the emotional challenges associated with pollen allergies and develop coping strategies to support your mental health. Consider the following tips for navigating emotional challenges:

1. Acknowledge Your Feelings: It's normal to feel frustrated, angry, or overwhelmed by the impact of pollen allergies on your life. Take time to acknowledge and validate your feelings, and give yourself permission to experience and express them without judgment.

2. Practice Self-Compassion: Be kind and compassionate toward yourself as you navigate the ups and downs of pollen allergy season. Treat yourself with the same understanding and care that you would offer to a loved one facing similar challenges.

3. Seek Emotional Support: Reach out to trusted friends, family members, or mental health professionals for emotional support and guidance. Sharing your experiences with others who understand can provide validation, comfort, and perspective.

4. Engage in Stress-Relieving Activities: Incorporate stress-relieving activities into your daily routine to promote relaxation and emotional well-being. Activities such as mindfulness meditation, yoga, deep breathing exercises, and spending time in nature can help reduce stress and improve mood.

5. Focus on What You Can Control: While you may not be able to control pollen levels or the onset of allergy symptoms, you can control how you respond to them. Focus on implementing practical strategies for managing your allergies and finding relief, rather than dwelling on factors beyond your control.

By acknowledging your feelings, practicing self-compassion, seeking emotional support, engaging in stress-relieving activities, and focusing on what you can control, you can navigate the emotional challenges of pollen allergy season with greater resilience and self-awareness.

COMMUNICATING WITH FAMILY, FRIENDS, AND CO-WORKERS

Effective communication is key to managing pollen allergies and maintaining healthy relationships with family, friends, and co-workers. Clear and open communication can help others understand your needs and limitations, reduce misunderstandings, and foster empathy and support. Consider the following tips for communicating about your allergies:

1. Educate Others: Take the time to educate your family, friends, and co-workers about pollen allergies, including common symptoms, triggers, and management strategies. Provide information about how allergies impact your daily life and what others can do to support you.

2. Be Honest and Direct: Be honest and direct about your needs and limitations due to pollen allergies. Clearly communicate any allergy triggers, dietary restrictions, or medication needs to ensure others are aware and can accommodate them when necessary.

3. Set Boundaries: Establish clear boundaries with others regarding activities or environments that may exacerbate your allergies. It's okay to decline invitations to outdoor events or ask for accommodations in indoor spaces to minimize your exposure to pollen.

4. Express Gratitude: Express gratitude to those who support and accommodate your allergies, whether it's by preparing allergy-friendly meals, providing emotional support, or making accommodations in shared spaces. Thank you could pass a protracted manner in fostering goodwill and strengthening relationships.

5. Be Patient and Understanding: Recognize that not everyone may fully understand or appreciate the impact of pollen allergies on your life. Be patient and understanding when answering questions or addressing concerns, and be open to providing additional information or clarification as needed.

By fostering open and honest communication with family, friends, and co-workers, you can cultivate understanding, empathy, and support for your pollen allergy management efforts.

Finding Support Groups and Resources

Connecting with others who share similar experiences can provide invaluable support and validation during pollen allergy season. Support groups and resources dedicated to pollen allergies can offer a sense of community, practical advice, and encouragement to help you cope with the challenges of allergy season. Consider the following options for finding support:

1. Online Support Groups: Join online forums, social media groups, or virtual support communities dedicated to pollen allergies. These platforms provide a space to connect with others, share experiences, ask questions, and offer support and encouragement.

2. Local Allergy Support Groups: Check for local allergy support groups or organizations in your area that host meetings, events, or educational programs for individuals with pollen allergies. Connecting with others face-to-face can provide a sense of belonging and camaraderie.

3. Allergy Education and Advocacy Organizations: Explore allergy education and advocacy organizations such as the Asthma and Allergy Foundation of America (AAFA) or Allergy UK, which provide resources, information, and support for individuals with allergies and their families.

4. Healthcare Providers and Allergy Specialists: Consult with your healthcare provider or allergy specialist for recommendations on local support groups, resources, or educational materials related to pollen allergies. They may be able to connect you with relevant resources or refer you to allergy-specific programs or services.

5. Educational Materials and Websites: Explore educational materials, books, websites, and online resources dedicated to pollen allergies. These resources may offer valuable information, tips, and strategies for managing allergies and finding relief.

By actively seeking out support groups and resources dedicated to pollen allergies, you can find solidarity, guidance, and encouragement from others who understand the challenges you face.

Living with pollen allergies presents unique challenges that require a multifaceted approach to management. By implementing coping strategies for emotional challenges, communicating effectively with others, and seeking support from support groups and resources, you can navigate pollen allergy season with greater resilience and confidence. Remember that you are not alone in your journey, and there are many resources and communities available to support you along the way. With patience, understanding, and self-care, you can find relief from pollen allergy symptoms and enjoy a healthier, more fulfilling life, even during allergy season.

Chapter 8: Thriving During Pollen Season

Pollen season can pose challenges for individuals with allergies, but with the right strategies and mindset, it's possible not just to survive but to thrive during this time of year. In this chapter, we'll explore how to enjoy outdoor activities safely, travel tips for allergy sufferers, and maintaining overall wellness to ensure you make the most of pollen season.

Enjoying Outdoor Activities Safely

For many people, pollen season coincides with warmer weather and the urge to spend more time outdoors. However, for allergy sufferers, outdoor activities can sometimes come with the risk of triggering allergy symptoms. Here are some tips for enjoying outdoor activities safely during pollen season:

1. Choose the Right Time: Pollen levels are typically highest in the early morning and early evening. Plan outdoor activities for midday when pollen levels are lower to minimize exposure.

2. Check Pollen Counts: Before heading outdoors, check local pollen counts using online resources or mobile apps. Avoid spending extended periods outdoors on days when pollen counts are high.

3. Wear Protective Clothing: When spending time outdoors, wear long-sleeved shirts, pants, sunglasses, and a wide-brimmed hat to minimize skin and eye contact with pollen.

4. Use Pollen-Blocking Accessories: Consider using pollen-blocking accessories such as nasal filters or masks when gardening or engaging in outdoor activities during peak pollen season.

5. Take Allergy Medication Beforehand: If you know you'll be spending time outdoors during pollen season, consider taking allergy medication beforehand to prevent symptoms from occurring.

By taking these precautions, you can reduce your risk of allergy symptoms and enjoy outdoor activities safely during pollen season.

Traveling Tips for Allergy Sufferers

Traveling during pollen season can present additional challenges for allergy sufferers, especially when visiting areas with different pollen profiles or environmental conditions. Here are some tips for traveling safely and comfortably during pollen season:

1. Research Your Destination: Before traveling, research the pollen levels and allergen triggers at your destination. Consider choosing destinations with lower pollen counts or visiting during times when pollen levels are typically lower.

2. Pack Allergy Essentials: Pack allergy essentials such as allergy medication, nasal sprays, eye drops, and tissues to have on hand during your trip. Consider bringing a travel-sized air purifier or allergy-proof bedding for added comfort.

3. Stay Indoors During High Pollen Times: Plan indoor activities or sightseeing during times when pollen levels are highest to minimize exposure. Seek out indoor attractions such as museums, galleries, or theaters to avoid pollen exposure.

4. Choose Allergy-Friendly Accommodations: When booking accommodations, consider choosing allergy-friendly options such as allergy-proof rooms or hotels with HEPA air filters to minimize allergen exposure.

5. Stay Hydrated and Rested: Traveling can be exhausting, especially for allergy sufferers. Stay hydrated, get plenty of rest, and listen to your body's cues to avoid overexertion and exacerbating allergy symptoms.

By planning ahead and taking proactive measures, you can enjoy your travels while minimizing the impact of pollen allergies on your trip.

MAINTAINING OVERALL WELLNESS

In addition to managing allergy symptoms, it's essential to prioritize overall wellness during pollen season to ensure you feel your best. Here are some tips for maintaining wellness:

1. Eat a Balanced Diet: Maintain a balanced diet rich in fruits, vegetables, whole grains, lean protein sources, and healthy fats to support immune function and overall health.

2. Stay Active: Regular physical activity can help boost immunity, reduce stress, and improve overall well-being. Find activities you enjoy and incorporate them into your daily routine, even during pollen season.

3. Practice Stress Management: Stress can exacerbate allergy symptoms and weaken the immune system. Practice stress management techniques such as mindfulness meditation, deep breathing exercises, or yoga to promote relaxation and emotional well-being.

4. Get Plenty of Sleep: Adequate sleep is essential for immune function and overall health. Aim for 7-9 hours of quality sleep per night to support your body's natural healing process.

5. Stay Connected: Maintain social connections with friends, family, and support networks to foster a sense of belonging and community. Share your experiences, seek support when needed, and offer support to others in return.

By prioritizing overall wellness, you can support your body's ability to cope with pollen allergies and enjoy a healthier, more fulfilling life, even during pollen season.

Pollen season may present challenges for allergy sufferers, but with the right strategies and mindset, it's possible not just to survive but to thrive during this time of year. By enjoying outdoor activities safely, following travel tips for allergy sufferers, and prioritizing overall wellness, you can make the most of pollen season and embrace the opportunities it brings. Remember to take care of yourself, listen to your body's cues, and seek support when needed. With patience, resilience, and a positive outlook, you can navigate pollen season with confidence and enjoy all that life has to offer.

CONCLUSION: EMPOWERING YOURSELF TO BREAK FREE FROM POLLEN ALLERGY SEASON

As we come to the end of this journey through pollen allergy season, it's essential to reflect on the strategies, tips, and insights shared throughout this book. Pollen allergies can be challenging to navigate, but by empowering yourself with knowledge, support, and practical tools, you can break free from the limitations imposed by allergy season and embrace a life of greater wellness and vitality.

Throughout this book, we've explored a wide range of topics, from understanding pollen allergies and identifying triggers to managing symptoms, seeking support, and thriving despite the challenges of pollen season. Each chapter has offered valuable insights and actionable strategies to help you take control of your allergies and live your life to the fullest. Let's take a moment to recap some of the key takeaways:

Understanding Pollen Allergies: We began our journey by delving into the fundamentals of pollen allergies, exploring what pollen is, how allergies develop, and common symptoms to watch out for. By understanding the underlying mechanisms of pollen allergies, you can better navigate pollen season and take proactive steps to manage your symptoms effectively.

Identifying Your Triggers: In Chapter 1, we explored the various types of pollen allergens, seasonal patterns, and allergic cross-reactivity that can impact allergy symptoms. By recognizing your unique allergy triggers, you can make informed choices about lifestyle modifications, allergy management strategies, and environmental precautions to minimize exposure and reduce symptoms.

Diagnosis and Testing: Chapter 2 highlighted the importance of consulting with healthcare professionals and undergoing allergy testing to accurately diagnose pollen allergies and develop a personalized treatment plan. By understanding the various testing options available and interpreting test results effectively, you can work with your healthcare team to identify the most appropriate treatments for your specific allergy needs.

Managing Pollen Exposure: In Chapter 3, we explored practical strategies for reducing pollen exposure both indoors and outdoors, from implementing allergy-friendly home environment tips to utilizing pollen forecasting and monitoring tools. By creating a supportive environment that minimizes allergen exposure, you can enjoy greater comfort and relief from allergy symptoms year-round.

Medications and Treatments: Chapter 4 delved into the various medications and treatments available for pollen allergies, including over-the-counter and prescription options, as well as immunotherapy. By exploring the benefits and considerations of each treatment approach, you can make informed decisions about which options may be most suitable for managing your allergies effectively.

Lifestyle Modifications: In Chapter 5, we discussed the importance of lifestyle modifications for pollen allergy relief, including creating an allergy-friendly home environment, making dietary considerations, and practicing stress management techniques. By incorporating these lifestyle changes into your daily routine, you can support your body's natural defenses and reduce the impact of pollen allergies on your life.

Natural Remedies and Alternative Therapies: Chapter 6 explored the use of herbal supplements, acupuncture, acupressure, and breathing exercises as complementary approaches to managing pollen allergy symptoms. By exploring natural remedies and alternative therapies, you can expand your toolkit for allergy relief and explore holistic approaches to wellness.

Coping Strategies and Support: Chapter 7 focused on coping strategies for navigating emotional challenges, communicating effectively with others about your allergies, and finding support groups and resources to help you cope with pollen allergy season. By fostering open communication, seeking support, and prioritizing self-care, you can navigate pollen season with greater resilience and confidence.

Thriving During Pollen Season: Finally, in Chapter 8, we explored how to thrive during pollen season by enjoying outdoor activities safely, traveling tips for allergy sufferers, and maintaining overall wellness. By embracing proactive strategies and a positive mindset, you can make the most of pollen season and enjoy a vibrant, fulfilling life, even in the face of allergy challenges.

As you embark on your journey beyond the pages of this book, remember that you are not alone in your struggle with pollen allergies. Reach out to healthcare professionals, support networks, and online communities for guidance, encouragement, and solidarity. By empowering yourself with knowledge, seeking support when needed, and embracing proactive strategies for allergy management, you can break free from the limitations imposed by pollen allergy season and live your life with vitality and joy.

So go ahead, step outside, breathe in the fresh air, and embrace the beauty of the world around you. With the right tools, support, and mindset, you have the power to thrive during pollen allergy season and beyond. Empower yourself, take control of your health, and embrace a life of wellness and possibility. The journey begins now.

Appendix: Resources

In this appendix, you'll find valuable resources to supplement your journey towards managing pollen allergies effectively. From a glossary of terms to help you navigate allergy-related terminology to allergy-friendly recipes that support your dietary needs, these resources aim to provide additional support and guidance as you navigate pollen allergy season and beyond.

Glossary of Terms

Understanding allergy-related terminology is essential for effectively communicating with healthcare professionals, interpreting medical information, and making informed decisions about allergy management.

This glossary of terms provides definitions for commonly used allergy terms and terminology:

1. Allergen: A substance that triggers an allergic reaction in individuals who are sensitive or allergic to it, such as pollen, dust mites, pet dander, or certain foods.

2. Allergic Rhinitis: Also known as hay fever, allergic rhinitis is an allergic reaction that occurs when the immune system overreacts to allergens such as pollen, causing symptoms such as sneezing, nasal congestion, itching, and watery eyes.

3. Antihistamine: A medication that blocks the action of histamine, a chemical released by the immune system in response to allergens, thereby reducing allergy symptoms such as sneezing, itching, and runny nose.

4. Immunotherapy: Also known as allergy shots or allergy immunotherapy, immunotherapy involves administering gradually increasing doses of allergens to desensitize the immune system and reduce allergic reactions over time.

5. Mast Cells: Cells of the immune system that release histamine and other inflammatory substances in response to allergen exposure, triggering allergic reactions

6. Nasal Steroid Spray: A medication administered via nasal spray that reduces inflammation in the nasal passages and relieves symptoms of allergic rhinitis such as nasal congestion, sneezing, and runny nose.

7. Peak Pollen Season: The time of year when pollen levels are highest, typically corresponding to the blooming season of specific plants or trees that produce pollen.

8. Sinusitis: Inflammation of the sinuses, often caused by viral or bacterial infections or underlying allergies, characterized by symptoms such as facial pain, headache, nasal congestion, and sinus pressure.

This glossary serves as a reference guide to help you navigate allergy-related terminology and enhance your understanding of pollen allergies and allergy management strategies.

ALLERGY-FRIENDLY RECIPES

Maintaining a balanced and nutritious diet is essential for supporting overall health and wellness, especially for individuals with pollen allergies. These allergy-friendly recipes are designed to be delicious, satisfying, and free from common allergens that may exacerbate allergy symptoms.

Whether you're looking for breakfast ideas, lunch options, or tasty treats, these recipes offer nutritious and flavorful meal options for individuals with pollen allergies:

1. Quinoa Breakfast Bowl: Start your day off right with a hearty quinoa breakfast bowl topped with fresh fruit, nuts, seeds, and a drizzle of honey or maple syrup for sweetness.
2. Allergy-Friendly Salad: Whip up a refreshing salad packed with leafy greens, colorful vegetables, protein-rich beans or tofu, and a homemade vinaigrette dressing for a nutritious and satisfying meal.
3. Roasted Vegetable Quinoa Salad: Combine roasted vegetables such as sweet potatoes, bell peppers, and zucchini with cooked quinoa, fresh herbs, and a tangy dressing for a flavorful and filling salad.
4. Allergy-Friendly Stir-Fry: Create a delicious stir-fry using your favorite vegetables, lean protein sources such as chicken or shrimp, and allergy-friendly sauces such as tamari or coconut aminos.
5. Banana-Oatmeal Cookies: Indulge your sweet tooth with these allergy-friendly banana-oatmeal cookies made with ripe bananas, oats, cinnamon, and a touch of honey or maple syrup for natural sweetness.
6. **Smoothie Bowl:** Blend up a nutrient-packed smoothie bowl with your favorite fruits, leafy greens, protein powder, and dairy-free milk for a refreshing and energizing meal or snack.

These allergy-friendly recipes offer nutritious and delicious meal options for individuals with pollen allergies, ensuring you can enjoy a varied and satisfying diet while managing your allergy symptoms effectively.

By utilizing these resources, you can enhance your understanding of pollen allergies, expand your culinary repertoire with allergy-friendly recipes, and take proactive steps towards managing your allergies and living a healthier, more fulfilling life. Remember to consult with healthcare professionals for personalized advice and guidance tailored to your individual allergy needs. With knowledge, support, and practical

POLLEN ALLERGY

46

POLLEN ALLERGY